I Beat Illness with FAITH

CANCER SURVIVOR

& YOU CAN TOO

I0442684

Copyright © 2020 by Brent Emmett Mandolph II
for NLV Publishing Company

All rights reserved. The use of any part of this publication reproduced, transmitted by any form or by any means, electronic, mechanical, photocopying, recording, or otherwise, or stored in a retrieval system, without the prior consent of the publisher is an infringement of the copyright law.

NLV Industries
4325 Glencoe Avenue
Unit 11594
Marina del Rey, CA 90295

213-293-6025 Direct
www.WinWithFaith.com

Cover Design: Brent Emmett Mandolph II
Book Layout: Brent Emmett Mandolph II

ISBN-13: 979-8550094297
ISBN-10: XXXXXXXXXX
BISAC: Medical / Healing
       Self-Help / Spiritual

Table of Contents

Table of Contents	*3*
I Beat Cancer with FAITH	*5*
— *"I WILL Beat Whatever They Say I Have!"*	
*The Letter **F** is for **FIGHT***	*11*
— You Must Decide to **FIGHT** for Your Recovery	
*The Letter **A** is for **ATTITUDE***	*19*
— You Must Maintain a Positive **ATTITUDE**	
*The Letter **I** is for **INSPIRATION***	*27*
— You Must Find a Source of **INSPIRATION**	
*The Letter **T** is for **TIME***	*35*
— You Must Give Yourself **TIME** to Recover	
*The Letter **H** is for **HELP***	*41*
— You Must Have **HELP** to Beat Cancer	
Epilogue	*49*
— You Can Beat Cancer with **FAITH** Too!!!	
Cancer Fighting Resources	*53*
— A Special Offer for the Reader	
— The Four (4) Fundamental Truths of Your Recovery	
— A Personal Message for the Reader	

I Beat Cancer with FAITH

"I HAVE FOUGHT THE GOOD FIGHT..."
"I HAVE FOUGHT THE GOOD FIGHT, I HAVE FINISHED THE COURSE, I HAVE KEPT THE FAITH"

— 2 TIMOTHY 4:7

Christmas 2019 – 7 Years of Cancer Freedom

December 18th, 2019, as I am preparing to take the stage to offer this wisdom to a room filled with cancer patients, survivors and doctors, I have just received the results of my most recent P.E.T Scan. The test has confirmed once again that I AM still cancer free. Considering my original prognosis, it is totally amazing that these tests have been confirming my cancer free status for more than 7 years now.

What great news to get as we head into the height of the holiday season with Christmas just one week away. This is the seventh Christmas that I will be celebrating with my family since falling out on that bus on that July morning in 2012, with what turned out to be bone marrow cancer – Multiple Myeloma, to be exact.

It's truly a miracle of FAITH that I am still here enjoying my family and friends, here to enjoy the first Christmas that my first grandchild is old enough to have some concept of the joy of the season. It has been an absolute pleasure to witness his reaction to everything from the Christmas decorations around town to the Christmas lights, or *"Kissmas Whites"* as he calls them, as we move around town.

To think that I could have easily not been here to witness any of this had I not had the FAITH to stand up to the dire situation that I found myself in. **God** only knows where I would be today if I hadn't had the power of FAITH to FIGHT back against cancer.

"I WILL Beat Whatever They Say I Have!"

July 14, 2012 – This is the day that my illness story began. It came upon me suddenly, seemingly out of nowhere. One day I was healthy and vibrant, and the next, I was lying flat on my back in a hospital bed, unable to sit up, roll over, and nowhere near able to stand up and walk.

I had just been hit with a medical crisis that delivered the worst pain I had ever felt in my life and knocked me totally off of my feet. To be sure, this was definitely a scary position to find myself in at just 46 years of age.

On that day, I had no clue of what had just landed in my life. Given the fact the pain seem to be coming from my chest, I personally thought that I was experiencing a heart attack. But the paramedics responding to my call for help quickly said it wasn't a heart attack.

I thought it could be some kind of a diabetic episode. After all, I did love my sugary donuts. But when my blood profile came in, I was quickly told that my blood sugar levels were excellent and I was nowhere near diabetic.

For most of us, there's nothing scarier than being hit with the words, *"You Have Cancer."* And, as this moment was playing out, that was the last thing that I thought I'd hear a doctor say to me.

Yet in some respects, it really didn't matter what I was diagnosed with because 17 years earlier, on another July day, the **Creator** had gifted me with a formula for APPLYING the power of FAITH to the crises that find their way into the path of life. Just having this wisdom in my possession had made me a fighter.

By now, 9 doctors had begun their work of trying to figure out what was going on inside of me, in earnest. As for me, I was worry free and in a place of peace. In large part, I was able to rest in this moment because I had been warned 8 years earlier that this day was coming.

I had been successfully using the wisdom of how to APPLY FAITH to the affairs of my life and overcoming great adversities for some years up to that point. Then the **Creator** whispered to me that the formula that was allowing me to win those battles was actually given to me for a yet to arrive day – a day when having a grasp on how to wield the power of FAITH would be vital to my life.

As I lay in my hospital room, waiting to find out what was ailing me, that little voice came back to me and told me that the problem that was rearing its head at that moment had already been answered. Then the principles that made up the FAITH formula were flashed on the screen of my mind. I knew what the message of that moment was.

As I reflected upon the big victories that that FAITH formula had brought me in the past, I KNEW that I could definitely handle this crisis as well. So on the strength of the FAITH power I KNEW I had at my disposal, I began to formulate the thought of getting my health back no matter what.

Out of this confidence, as I sat there still not knowing what was ailing me, I preemptively decided that *"I WOULD BEAT WHATEVER THE DOCTORS CAME BACK AND SAID I HAD."* And, though I didn't know it at the time, making the declaration that I would *"BEAT"* whatever the doctors diagnosed me with is likely what saved my life.

Admittedly, having had the experience of hearing a doctor speak the words *"YOU HAVE CANCER,"* I can say that the moment is definitely a surreal one. It seems like in a blur you go from being well, to being confronted by some troubling symptoms, to waiting for answers to what's ailing you, to finding out that your worst nightmare has come true, *"You Have Cancer."*

For most people, just hearing those words is like being given a literal death sentence. At that moment, the programmed response may be to ask the doctor, *"How much time do I have?"* And, unfortunately, too many doctors are perfectly willing to answer this ill-conceived question.

To begin with, the patient asking is usually not in the best state of mind to handle such a weighty discussion. And sadly, for far too many people confronted with this crisis, it never occurs at that moment that all illness can be fought and all illness can be beat.

I know these things to be true because I have already had to face each one of them. When I was confronted with that surreal moment, fortunately everything was totally different.

I had a firm grasp on how to wield the power of FAITH and the **God** given, 8 principle formula that would help me unleash that power on this developing crisis. I also KNEW not to ask that question and was blessed to have a wonderful doctor who never even tried to hold that discussion.

Instead, we began our work together by discussing my FAITH, he literally inquired about my level of FAITH with the very first words he spoke to me. Then he moved to offer assurance that the malady that he was about to lay squarely at my feet was fightable, a perfect beginning considering that I had already committed myself to fighting and winning before I even KNEW who or what my opponent was.

Today, more than 7 years later, sitting here as a last stage cancer survivor, I know beyond a shadow of a doubt that you can fight and beat illness. And, now having had the occasion to personally meet and interview 32 other survivors of all types of cancer, I know beyond all doubt that you can beat all manner of illness with FAITH.

I also know that when most people even think about fighting back against illness, they think about beefing up for the physical aspects of the fight. Or, they think about beefing up in the area of their diet and fitness regimen.

They even think about bolstering their immune systems. And there is nothing wrong with endeavoring to make those improvements. Even the doctors will advise their patients to endeavor in these ways.

But from my experience and observation, there's another vital area that is seldom thought about by the average patient or doctor, an area that few realize offers a proven path to healing – the area of our FAITH! Yet to a person, each one of the 32 cancer survivors that I have met said the development of their FAITH was among their highest priorities.

In fact, each of these men/women described FAITH power as one of the main elements of their victory over their illness and I agree. I agree because I not only beat illness, to be exact, I beat a Bone Marrow cancer with just one round of chemotherapy, one round of radiation and NO BONE MARROW TRANSPLANT. That's how I KNOW I BEAT illness with FAITH and YOU can too!!!

Using F.A.I.T.H. as an acronym let me share some of the working principles of FAITH that the **Creator** revealed to me when He gifted me with the wisdom of FAITH (APPLIED). Applying these principles to your battle with illness will allow you to activate the kind of FAITH that has allowed me and others to beat a major illness.

The letter "F" is for FIGHT

"FIGHT THE GOOD FIGHT OF FAITH..."
"FIGHT THE GOOD FIGHT OF FAITH; TAKE HOLD OF THE ETERNAL LIFE TO WHICH YOU WERE CALLED AND YOU MADE THE GOOD CONFESSION IN THE PRESENCE OF MANY WITNESSES."
— 1 TIMOTHY 6:12

Before you can beat illness, you have to make up your mind to FIGHT it. And, perhaps before you can truly make up your mind to FIGHT back against illness, you need to know that you can.

So much of our society considers the major illnesses as un-fightable diseases — as literal death sentences for anyone who is unfortunate enough to have one barge its way into their life.

While it is certainly true that people die of major illnesses, the fact is that many people FIGHT and beat them. Since I beat the cancer that barged its way into my life more than 7 years ago, I have personally met 32 other people who have done the same.

These men and women were from all backgrounds, all ages, all races and had various cancers. While there really are no junior cancers, some have fought and defeated illnesses that are often thought of as simply UNBEATABLE!

What I learned talking with these men/women was that aside from a strong belief in the power of FAITH, we all shared one thing in common. We were willing to FIGHT back against the illness that had attacked our bodies.

Now I know that sounds simplistic. And I also know how easy it is to assume that everyone who is stricken with an illness FIGHTS it. I used to think the same thing before I was diagnosed. But from my experience I can now say that it's just not true.

For a variety of reasons, some people who are attacked by a major disease never step up to FIGHT it. As I have said, I have already personally met 32 other cancer survivors. And, I have also met an equal or perhaps even a greater number of people who unfortunately had their lives cut short by illness.

Just as the survivors I met all shared key traits in common, those I met who lost their battle with illness also shared key things in common. One of those things was a spoken unwillingness to FIGHT to beat the disease and to live.

That unwilling spirit was rooted in many factors: misinformation, fear, lack of FAITH, little or NO support, bad doctors, to name a few. But whatever its roots, the fact is none of us can win a FIGHT against illness that we never undertake. I know again that this seems like a given, but I am telling you that it really is not.

You have to make up in your mind that **YOU ARE GOING TO FIGHT THE ILLNESS THAT IS IN FRONT OF YOU**.

In fact, affirm this out loud right now:

I AM FIGHTING YOU ILLNESS!!!

I AM GOING TO FIGHT YOU AND I AM GOING TO BEAT YOU, NO MATTER WHAT YOUR NAME IS!!!

Say that! And, as you do, know that the **Creator** has not only given you the authority and right to do so. He has also given you the victory over that illness at the very moment that you **"Accept the Challenge"** of taking that illness on.

Scripture says that, *"Death and Life are in the power of the tongue..."* Proverbs 18:21

That means that you have the right and power to speak life or death to your life. That also means that you are speaking life or death to your life with the words that you choose to speak.

As you look out at this health challenge that lies before you, if you want to beat it, you must become conscious of the language that you and everyone around you uses in relationship to the situation.

If you want to beat it, you must begin to speak life and only life to your situation. You should never even contemplate the disease beating you and certainly not your death.

Every cancer survivor that I have met, including me said they did these two things habitually – spoke only victory and life; and they never considered their death. Speaking for me, I didn't slip in either of these ways for even 1 second of my recovery process.

Also, scripture says that, *"The Lord, Heals all our diseases..."* Psalms 103:3

It also says that, *"This sickness is not unto death, but for the glory of **God**, that the Son of **God** might be glorified through it."* John 11:4

That means that if you can have FAITH and take the **Creator** at his word, you already have the assurance of victory, even before you begin your FIGHT. So now will you FIGHT?

*If the **Creator** is for you, who or what can truly be against you?* Romans 8:31 poses that question then goes on to demonstrate that the only answer you and I can have is, "NO ONE & NOTHING!"

So now that you know that you can FIGHT, should FIGHT and that the **Creator** has already given you the victory, let me give you two specific things that you must FIGHT against.

1. You Must FIGHT the illness Itself

It bears repeating that for you to beat that illness, you have got to go to war against it. More than anything else, that means that you have to commit to getting yourself to the doctor and after consultation, running the game plan for your recovery.

It means taking the medicines, treatments and procedures prescribed in that plan and giving them a chance to do their job. It means staying engaged and committed even when the process gets painful and uncomfortable.

I get to say that to you because I did it myself. I have to say it because this seemingly simple thing is where I watched many of the people who I know that lost their battle blow it.

The plain truth is that this is the front line of your FIGHT with any illness. It is ground zero and the vigor with which you attack here will determine whether or not you win your FIGHT against illness.

To be clear, when I say that *"I Beat illness With FAITH!"* by no means do I wish to convey the notion that I beat that illness without doctors, medicines, treatment regiments or procedures. By no means am I trying to suggest that I had no relationship to TRADITIONAL WESTERN MEDICINE. Again, this is where I have seen many people blow it.

Whether out of fear, ignorance or plain stupidity, those people who I knew who failed to see the wisdom in working with a doctor lost their FIGHT against illness. Most often they failed to avail themselves of the medical resources that likely could have saved their life. Even some big name public figures of our time did the same thing.

In the end, most of the ones I knew expressed deep regret at not doing so just before their passing. Don't you do it! As the **Creator** told me as I lay in the back of the ambulance that was taking me to the hospital to begin my FIGHT, *"TAKE YOUR BUTT TO THE DOCTOR!"* It's there that you do most of your physical FIGHTING.

Take advantage of their wisdom and expertise. Be thankful that you live in a time where the luxury of health care is readily available. The same thing goes for the medicines, treatments and procedures.

Be grateful for them. Give a prayer of thanks for their availability. Ask the **Creator** to prepare your body, mind and spirit to receive their healing benefits.

Then know that He is doing just that. That's what I did! And, guess what? It worked! I Beat illness with these FAITH principles and I know that You Can Too!!!

Now I must say that when I first was stricken with cancer, I thought that all I had to do was beat the illness itself and then I'd be able to return to life as I knew it before. I now know, just as all other survivors do that that is just not how it works. To totally whip illness, you have to also take on this next FIGHT.

2. You Must FIGHT the Aftermath of the illness

To truly win your FIGHT against illness, you have to also take on and defeat any/all of the issues that crop up in the aftermath of your bout. In my case, the battle with active cancer was a relatively short one and in no time I started getting good reports of clean blood test and scans that looked to see if I had any active cancer in my body.

Starting out on the road to recovery, I would have thought that those positive results meant, *"Mission Accomplished!"* But that just wasn't the truth. Far and away for me, the longest FIGHT has been with the aftermath of the battle – the condition that illness and being off my feet for so long left my body in, the side effects of the medicines, treatments and the procedures that I had to undertake to return to health.

Dealing with the *"New Normals"* that have resulted from the impairments and scars left from the battle, plus the ways in which my body and life has changed temporarily. That has been a FIGHT in its own right.

The FIGHT now is to return to regular life and to keep these changes from becoming permanent. These two have been the fronts upon which I have had to FIGHT against illness. In telling you this truth, it's my hope to prepare you fully for the FIGHT that is standing in front of you.

I'm endeavoring to get you ready for battle. I'm trying to paint an accurate and clear picture of the enemy to your health that you are about to take down.

Here again, I can assure you that you have the victory even before you start out in the FIGHT, especially because we are getting you ready for the real and full battle. For sure I have gained a victory over the *"Aftermath"* and I wasn't aware of this battlefront.

While there is still some mop up work to be done in my health and fitness levels, I can assure you that not only did I not experience all of the bad side effects that are so often feared. I can also tell you that the ones I did experience have all just about cleared up over time.

I know that it will work out the same way for you, if you will give it a FIGHTING chance. I also believe that just having the awareness that you'll need to FIGHT on both of these fronts will give you the mental and emotional stamina that you will need to *"Beat"* illness.

So have you made a firm decision to FIGHT and BEAT the illness that is in front of you? Declare your victory right now before the world! Affirm these declarations out loud:

> ### FAITH Declaration #1
> *– I AM going to BEAT this illness!!!*
>
> ### FAITH Declaration #2
> *– I AM going to BEAT this illness's AFTERMATH!!!*

In the spirit of Proverbs 18:21 learn to *"Speak life to your life"* and life is what you'll receive. Say them again and again out loud! Affirm them everyday to get it deep inside of you!

Now let's look at the next powerful letter in our F.A.I.T.H. acronym.

The letter "A" is for ATTITUDE

"I 'Can Do' all things..."
"I can do all things through Christ who strengthens me."
— Philippians 4:13

When it comes to beating illness, ATTITUDE IS EVERYTHING! As you FIGHT, you may have enough to deal with just getting through the average day. Your day will be made all the more challenging if you approach it in the wrong spirit or with a bad ATTITUDE.

When it comes to having the type of ATTITUDE that will get you by illness, it's a must that we first talk about the power of the **"Can Do"** ATTITUDE. Possessing an ATTITUDE that says **"I Can Beat Illness"** is the starting point to you beating illness.

To be sure, I brought the "Can Do" spirit to my FIGHT against multiple myeloma – the illness that attacked me. I guess it was easy for me to tap into this ATTITUDE because I had a full understanding of the "Can Do" power of FAITH before illness barged into my life.

In fact, I had used a **God** given formula for FAITH to take on the challenges that had been thrown into my life's path for 17 years prior to cancer. That time and those victories had given me a deep confidence in what my **God** given FAITH could do to rescue me from any and all crises.

As scripture says, I knew that, *"I 'Can Do' all things through Christ who strengthens me."* Philippians 4:13

I was confident that with the better than *"Mustard Seed of FAITH"* that existed within me I would be able to *"Move the*

Mountain" of cancer and that I would *"Do the Impossible"* of beating it and the paralysis that came with it, just as Matthew 17:20 said I could.

Having this level of FAITH at the beginning of my battle against illness allowed me to be positive from the outset of the FIGHT. And looking back now, this positive ATTITUDE was vital to my ability to find healing.

I instinctively knew that I needed to maintain a positive, upbeat ATTITUDE and keep my spirits up no matter how dire the situation might have looked. And, because I knew the power of FAITH and because I knew the faithfulness of the **Creator**, I found it easy to keep my spirits high as I worked through this scary moment in my life.

In fact scripture says, *"Keep your mind on things that are above, not on things that are on the earth."* Colossians 3:2

That means that to keep your spirits up and your ATTITUDE right, you must set your mind and heart on the things above. You must set your mind and heart on the healing promises of **God** and not the fact that you've been diagnosed with an illness – even if the prognosis isn't a favorable one.

Perhaps you need to do this even more so when the outlook for your victory or survival isn't that good. That's what I did. I never dealt in the diagnosis or the prognosis while I was actively fighting cancer.

Instead I purposely chose to look through the lens of positivity out at a future in which I would be healed and my good health restored. Every survivor that I know maintained a similar outlook. If you will do the same, you too will *"Keep your mind off the things that are on earth,"* like I did.

With the help of my wife, a large part of how I did it was to control my environment. Starting with my hospital room, we set up an environment that was totally about my healing. We controlled which people got access to me. And, it didn't matter who they were.

I never would have dreamed of having to throw doctors and nurses out of my midst, but it happened. For us, it didn't matter that these were supposedly medical professionals.

The fact was that if they had a negative ATTITUDE, if they didn't believe like I did concerning my healing they were not there to help me heal. So that meant that even these medical experts had to go.

As scripture teaches, *"Do not be yoked together with unbelievers..."* 2 Corinthians 6:14

In controlling my environment in this way, we seriously controlled who had the ability to affect my ATTITUDE. In fact, when I was in the hospital, we built such a positive atmosphere and I was generally in such an excellent mood that several of my nurses made my room their lounge.

They literally took their breaks and lunches with me and we talked about everything but the illness that I was fighting to beat. It was truly a testament to the ATTITUDE and demeanor that I was in. As far as I am concerned, there is no way to FIGHT a serious illness with an ATTITUDE that is filled with negativity.

Additionally, my spirits were helped by the fact that my family totally allowed me to leave the cares of this world behind me while I endeavored to beat the illness that attacked me. I know that a large part of what allowed me to win my FIGHT was the positive ATTITUDE that I was able to keep up throughout my FIGHT as a result.

Scripture says, *"A cheerful heart is good medicine, but a crushed spirit dries up the bones!"* Proverbs 17:22

I noticed that along with me, every other one of the 32 survivors that I met had a cheerful spirit. And sadly, every one of the people that I personally knew who lost their battle against major illness had a negative one, the exact opposite.

From what I could see, they had the habit of counting every *"Ouch"* that they experienced. When considering their future, they also generally had a fatalistic outlook.

It's certainly understandable why they would feel the way they did. To be sure, being confronted with a diagnosis of a serious illness, dealing with all that you have to go through because of it and looking out into an uncertain future is a lot to take in for anyone.

But the fact still remains that you have to stay positive. You have to realize that it really is a classic *"Glass half full or glass half empty"* circumstance. I know that I was able to maintain my positive ATTITUDE because I have always been a *"Glass half full"* type of person.

I have always been the type of person that is able to look at the positive side of things, no matter what circumstance I find myself in. That trait perfectly lines up with the scripture that says,

"Brothers and sisters, whatever is true, whatever is noble, whatever is right, whatever is pure, whatever is lovely,

whatever is admirable – if anything is excellent or praiseworthy – think about such things." Philippians 4:8

Decide that you are going to keep a great positive, healing ATTITUDE!!! No matter where you are in the recovery process. I know that this positive, healing ATTITUDE is a large part of what saved my life. And I know that if you will adopt and maintain this ATTITUDE it will save your life too. Just as I know that if you will always strive to see the glass as *"Half Full"* you will come through this challenging moment with flying colors.

Keep a Good ATTITUDE with Uplifting Entertainment

There was one other tool I used to maintain the positive ATTITUDE that helped me beat illness, it was the power of **Uplifting Entertainment**. Whether it was music from the old days, television programs or movies, I totally indulged myself with this material and all of the good vibes and memories that it brought back to me.

Whether it was to keep me laughing, hopeful or inspired, I used the power of this spirit lifting resource to keep my ATTITUDE up while I was engaged in the FIGHT against multiple myeloma. I reached back in time and immersed myself in this entertainment of my childhood and through it I was able to totally take my mind off of all of the weighty matters that were in front of me.

On several occasions, this content helped me to escape from the harsh realities of my FIGHT against cancer. By keeping these images in front of me on a regular basis, I was able to keep my spirits upbeat and my ATTITUDE in a good place.

Overall I was able to keep my spirits high throughout the time I was in active treatment for multiple myeloma. However, there were a few times during the thick of my battle with this deadly illness that I found myself in a down and dark place.

At those moments, I had let the reality that illness had attacked my body get to me. On those occasions, I literally had to put on entertainment like holiday movies to lift my spirits up out of the dark mood that I had fallen into.

On one such occasion, this spirit came upon me when I was at home by myself, in need of help with a simple task that I used to easily handle. At that moment I was confronted with my newly formed physical impairments and it got the best of me emotionally. It took losing myself in the classic holiday movie *"Elf"* to redirect my emotions and lift my ATTITUDE back up.

I usually kept my mind fully off of the realities of my illness diagnosis and the challenges that resulted from it. I often used the resource of **Uplifting Entertainment** to do it.

I wasn't in denial. I just instinctively knew that there was no value in dwelling on all of the negative details of dealing with the disease confronting me.

One of the FAITH principles that I learned long before being diagnosed with cancer was the importance of *Delaying Judgment*. I knew that no matter how impossible the task may look, no matter how behind you appear to be in the FIGHT, if you can simply *Delay Judgment* and FIGHT on, you can turn the situation around in the end.

There's no way to *Delay Judgment* while you're in a dark place. It's also tough to keep up a good ATTITUDE when your mind is filled with all of the negative details of your predicament. And, it's easier to stay out of that dark place if you feed your mind with a constant supply of uplifting content.

I watched old TV programs and movies that I always enjoyed. I also listened to old music and used the internet to view concerts that I always enjoyed. Conversely, I consciously avoided viewing anything that could bring my spirits down.

I have no doubt that these seemingly little acts made a big difference in my ability to find healing. I know that if you'll make the effort to do these same things, it will help you to find healing to.

Develop an illness beating ATTITUDE

As you embark upon your FIGHT with illness, there have to be people that you can look to who are beating the disease and who can help you adopt the *"Can Do"* ATTITUDE that you will need to beat it too.

Now, to HELP you develop this *"Can Do"* spirit, list three people you know (or, know of) who have beat the illness confronting you (or who are currently beating it. Do research and find someone, if need be):

1._____
2._____
3._____

Next, each one of us has had an interest or hobby that has always brought us great joy. Perhaps we were forced to put it aside out of the busy-ness and obligations of life. And, perhaps rekindling it at this trying time could be a source of much needed joy – joy that can help you to maintain the positive and upbeat ATTITUDE that you need to beat that illness.

Now, list three steps you can take to rekindle an interest or hobby and bring that joy back to your life:

1._____
2._____
3._____

Lastly, nothing has the ability to keep your spirits and your ATTITUDE uplifted like the **Uplifting Entertainment** from your past.

So to tap into this power, list some music, movies and television shows that have always given you great joy and that you can turn to now in moments when you need a quick lift of your spirits and ATTITUDE:

1._____
2._____
3._____

Additionally, take the time to re-read this section. When you do, take special note of the concepts of *stepping away from the day to day cares of life, keeping a positive environment and a "Glass Half-Full" outlook, as well as "Delaying Judgment" on weighty issues*. Be sure to inject each one of these concepts into your world to keep your spirits lifted high and your ATTITUDE good.

Also, where you involve others in the handling of your personal and financial affairs, continue to sign your own checks and otherwise oversee everything related to your finances, if you can. Unfortunately, bad things often happen when you give over unchecked access to your money and your financial resources.

Don't you become a victim as you allow others to help you with simple day to day and financial tasks. Do these things and you are sure to reserve your energy and ATTITUDE for your efforts to beat the illness standing before you.

Now let's look at the next letter in our powerful F.A.I.T.H. acronym.

The letter "I" is for INSPIRATION

"INSPIRATION GIVES UNDERSTANDING..."

"BUT THERE IS A SPIRIT IN MAN: AND THE INSPIRATION OF THE ALMIGHTY GIVES THEM UNDERSTANDING."

— JOB 32:8

Fighting any great challenge gets a whole lot easier to do when you realize all that you have to FIGHT for, when you have a clear source of INSPIRATION or a "WHY" as it's often called. Fighting a major illness is no different.

To give yourself the power of one of the most basic sources of INSPIRATION, you can think about the family and friends you love and who love you. You can think of how these people still need you or how you still have unfinished business in their lives.

Many of the cancer survivors that I have met have told me expressly that they drew INSPIRATION to get through the tough times they had to endure fighting their illness from thinking about the impact their passing would have on their loved ones. Specifically, they thought about the plans and goals they wouldn't be here to accomplish if their illness had defeated them.

How would the lives of those you love the most be impacted if you were permanently incapacitated or gone? If you are old enough to have children or grandchildren, what about those yet to be born?

When I first fell ill, neither of my sons had become fathers yet. But that changed nearly 5 years later when my eldest had his first son, my first grandchild.

Today, my little grandson Legend is the delight of my life and a great source of INSPIRATION for me to keep on beating illness. His being here has made me dust off several goals and plans that I had put away when his dad and uncle became men. It also gave me several new dreams for his future.

To think that if I had not fought and beat illness, I would not have lived to see him born. I would not have lived to experience the joy of being a grandfather and to enjoy this time in my life.

No matter where you are in life there has to be someone in your life that is worth fighting and living for. That has to be true whether you are young or old. It's okay for you to draw INSPIRATION from that relationship!

In fact, it's said that *"we will do far more for the people that we love than we will for ourselves."* It's okay to draw the power to FIGHT from the things that you wanted to do for others that would go undone if illness beat you or took you away now – the goals and dreams that you had purposed for the people that you care about. It's okay to let this powerful source of motivation INSPIRE you.

Get INSPIRED by your own "Unfinished Business"

What about your own unfinished business? What about the personal goals and dreams that would be left undone if you were permanently defeated or left this life now?

What about the things that you wanted to accomplish with your own life, the mark you wanted to leave on the world to show you were here? What about your own legacy?

Another powerful source of INSPIRATION can be found in the plans that you had for your life that you are still working to complete. When I lay in that ambulance at the beginning of my illness moment I was consumed with the thought of my unfinished business.

In this moment that I now call my "NEAR, NEAR Death Experience," my mind was racing with all the things that I never completed; the goals and dreams that I had held dear for years. I was consumed with the thought that these long sought after plans would all go unfinished if I had passed away at that moment.

In that moment I actually thought that I was having a heart attack and was powerless to see these tasks through. But once I was told that I wasn't in danger of dying on the spot I promised myself that I would beat whatever illness was standing in the way of me going to get these accomplishments.

I then drew INSPIRATION to FIGHT cancer from those unfinished goals and dreams. Nearly every survivor that I have met told me they draw major power to FIGHT from the "WHY" of their unfinished business. I know you can draw major INSPIRATION from your unfinished business too.

It's said that, *"If we have a strong enough "WHY", we can endure almost any how."* I believe that is true. I hope that you will look around you and within you and consider all the reasons "WHY" you must beat that illness. Hopefully then you will BE INSPIRED TO FIGHT and BEAT ILLNESS!

You need the "RIGHT" kind of INFORMATION to beat illness

The letter "I" could have also easily been for INFORMATION! That's because a large part of you beating illness will be based upon what INFORMATION does and does not flow to you while you are engaged in the FIGHT.

To put it plain, you need all of the INFORMATION that is going to help you wage a successful war against the disease. In this way, knowledge is power and ignorance is a liability.

On the other hand, you don't need one grain of the kind of INFORMATION that points to your defeat. Where that kind of INFORMATION is concerned, ignorance is the source of power and knowledge is most often a huge liability.

You need to know about all of the medicines that are available to you and the full range of treatment options and procedures that can help you find healing and restoration. You don't need to know about all of the side effects that could occur in the healing process. And, you definitely don't need to know *"HOW MUCH TIME YOUR DOCTORS THINK YOU HAVE?"*

No matter what their level of experience or expertise, no doctor can definitively tell you that. What they can do by trying to tell you that is scare you into giving up and letting illness win or take you out without you putting up a serious FIGHT.

And I get to tell you that considering that back in July of 2012, 8 of the 9 doctors that greeted me when I first arrived at the hospital that treated me predicted that I would live no more than 6 months. I laugh every time I think about that today. I often tell people that by their count, I am 7 years old right now because I have now lived a full 7 years past their prediction.

Under most all circumstances, no one has the right, power or skill to predict your life expectancy. Again, scripture says that, *"Death and Life are in the power of YOUR tongue!"* It also says that **Jesus** has *"healed your illness!"* And it didn't make a distinction that excluded that illness from the illnesses that **Jesus** has healed you of.

If you must let some basic INFORMATION in regarding the illness you are fighting, let that in. But taking in all its negative attributes, or all the possible side effects fighting it may not even bring to you; or issues that will reverse themselves over time, will surely scare you into not taking it on.

This type of INFORMATION can only serve to make you hesitant to follow the treatment protocol that's prescribed to bring you **God's** gift of healing. Just as filling your mind with what could go wrong or predictions (guesses) about how your fight will turn out or how much longer you will be on the planet can only serve to discourage and scare you and those who truly love you.

Fortunately for me that 1 doctor who was willing to stand and FIGHT with me against illness, didn't INFORM me of his colleagues pessimistic outlook until I had beat it by 4 years. He disagreed with the prediction and took great pride in us proving them wrong.

That's why I know that you have to avoid anyone, doctors, family members, friends, even others with your same illness who want to engage you in such talk – and I mean ANYONE! There is no value in that type of INFORMATION.

Likewise, you don't need to talk about all of the negative side effects that might come from the medicines, treatments and procedures that you have to go through to find your healing. Personally, I never experienced most of the "Side Effects" that I heard come from things like taking Chemotherapy and Radiation treatments.

And, now 7 years later, I have recovered from all but one of the collateral challenges that did present themselves in the aftermath of my recovery. Thank **God** when I was in active treatment I didn't take in a bunch of INFORMATION regarding this matter.

Of course, for liability reasons, the medical team treating me had to cover these concerns and I had to sign waivers giving my consent to go ahead anyway. But each time I signed and didn't dwell on the INFORMATION. Instead I maintained my same upbeat demeanor and went forward in pursuit of healing, just as all of the other survivors I have met did.

So seek out the INSPIRATION and the INFORMATION that will allow you to beat that illness. Below take a moment to list your *"WHY"* – the people or unfinished goals and dreams that you can draw INSPIRATION from to beat illness.

"WHY" I must beat this illness & live!!

_____
_____
_____
_____
_____
_____
_____

_____
_____
_____
_____
_____
_____
_____
_____
_____
_____

Now let's look at the fourth letter in our powerful F.A.I.T.H. acronym.

The letter "T" is for TIME

"ENDURE TO THE END AND BE SAVED..."

"BUT HE THAT SHALL ENDURE UNTO THE END, THE SAME SHALL BE SAVED."

— MATTHEW 24:13

You must give yourself TIME to be healed and restored from illness. To be clear, your complete healing miracle will take TIME to manifest. By no means am I suggesting otherwise.

Most people think of being healed with FAITH as an instantaneous healing event. However, my healing didn't come in an instant. None of the other survivors that I met received their healing in an instant.

And, most likely you won't receive your healing miracle in an instant either. The fact is that even a healing miracle takes TIME, just as a FAITH manifestation takes TIME. But just because your healing takes TIME, doesn't mean that your healing isn't taking place.

You have to give yourself TIME to heal and for that matter, TIME to recover. In fact, you have to be patient and give yourself whatever amount of TIME it takes for you to heal and get back to the life you knew before illness barged into your life.

Scripture teaches us the importance of giving yourself TIME in a trying moment where it says,

"Be joyful in Hope, patient in Affliction and FAITHFUL in prayer." Romans 12:12

You will never stumble off of the path to healing and restoration if you remember those wise words.

In my book, **FAITH (APPLIED)**, I write about three TIME related stumbling blocks that I've seen trip folks up on their path to recovery. Teaching them to you now can make the difference between you beating illness and losing your good health or life to it.

Stumbling Block #1 – Failing to Realize You Must Beat the Disease and the Aftermath to Truly Beat illness!

We've already talked about this, but it bears repeating that to truly beat illness, you have to beat both the disease that has barged into your life and whatever aftermath comes from the sickness and all of the medicines, treatments and procedures that gave you your victory. When it comes to winning against a serious illness, that's the whole truth.

It's the, *"Not Knowing This"* that makes it a stumbling block. It's when you go into your FIGHT thinking all you have to do is beat the illness and you get hit by an aftermath so formidable that it makes you think you aren't beating the illness after all.

It's in that moment that this truth causes you to stumble off the path of recovery all together. Going into the FIGHT knowing who the real opponent is will keep you in the FIGHT when the battle front switches up from the actual disease to its aftermath.

Let's look at the next thing that can get in the way of recovery.

Stumbling Block #2 – Failing to Realize that Beating a Major illness is a Process, Not an Event!

The simple truth is that when it comes to healing and restoring your body and life back to the way it was before that illness, *"It is a Process, not an Event!"* In my case, it is more than 7 years later and I am still healing.

I am still seeing and experiencing new milestones in my recovery. And, I am still having abilities that I had lost return to me and my body.

As I have gone through the healing process, I have asked my doctors if the abilities that I had lost would return to me. None of them have ever been able to answer me with a definitive "Yes!" Under a cloud of uncertainty, I had to give myself TIME to find out the answer to my questions.

If I couldn't or wouldn't give myself that TIME, it would have been very easy to slip into frustration and doubt and the negative emotions that come as a result. In fact, the easiest way to let frustration and doubt creep in is for you to get impatient with the healing process.

That can't happen if you keep in mind that *healing is a process, not an event*. It's knowing that that will keep you from stumbling off the path of recovery. From my experience, going into the FIGHT knowing *"It's a process, not an event"* will keep you in the FIGHT for the long haul.

And, it's staying in the FIGHT that will give you the best chance of finding complete healing and restoration.

Let's look at the next thing that can get in the way of recovery.

Stumbling Block #3 – Failing to Realize You Must Earn Back the Health that illness Takes Away!

The truth is that illness may change the state of your physical health. It may make you weak. It may impair you. It may even disable you. When it does you have to work to earn back the state of wellness and mobility that you enjoyed before illness blindsided you.

If the the illness doesn't do it, the aftermath of all of the medicines, treatments and procedures that you will have to undertake to find your healing may. If it does, the hope of every survivor is that these changes are both minor and temporary.

That was my hope. At the height of my battle, I had to come back from both cancer and partial paralysis. I found myself flat on my back, stuck in the bed. I was totally unable to even roll over or sit up in the bed. And I wasn't able to even think about getting out of that bed.

That condition represented a drastic change from the body and the level of mobility that I knew before illness. Obviously, it represented a major battle to have to wage on top of the battle against the illness that put me in that position.

Given the severity of the changes I experienced in my body, it would have been easily justifiable for me to have felt like I'd never return back to the state of health and mobility I previously enjoyed. But fortunately I had the wisdom that I needed to work to earn back the level of health I once enjoyed, no matter how trying that task may have turned out to be.

Fortunately I knew I had to work my way back from this deadly illness and the crippling condition it brought with it. I had to stay in FAITH as I worked to comeback from these very serious health challenges.

Glory to **God**, I did get back on my feet. It took some EFFORT. To be exact, it took 6 months to get out of that bed and another 12 months to get back walking.

Once I got back on my feet the real FIGHT began, the FIGHT to earn back the mobility that this fight with illness took away from me. I had to give myself TIME to take up and win that FIGHT. And that's a FIGHT that I am still battling and winning gains in to this day.

The best way to insure that you handle each of these stumbling blocks is to give yourself TIME to recover. It bears repeating that it takes TIME for your doctors and the medicines, treatments and procedures they prescribe to take affect and do their work. It takes TIME to overcome all of the challenges this FIGHT will bring to your life and your body.

If you are serious about beating illness you must patiently give yourself whatever TIME it takes for you to recover. Will you pledge to give yourself that TIME? Take this *Survivor's TIME pledge for Healing* with me right now:

> ## *Survivor's TIME Pledge for Healing*
>
> *– I pledge to give myself ALL of the TIME it takes to heal & overcome the illness I'm fighting and the aftermath of that illness I must FIGHT!*
>
> *– I pledge to give myself this TIME to heal in a spirit of absolute FAITH, trusting that God will bring me through, fully healed – with my health fully restored, as He promised in His holy word!*

Come back to this pledge over and over until you get its message down deep in your heart. Then give yourself all of the TIME that you need to truly beat illness.

Now let's look at the final letter in our powerful F.A.I.T.H. acronym.

The letter "H" is for HELP

"Two are better than one..."

"Two are better than one, because they have a good return for their labor: If either of them falls down, one can help the other up. But pity anyone who falls and has no one to help them up."

— Ecclesiastes 4:9-10

You need HELP to beat illness. The plain truth is that NO ONE beats a serious illness alone. I and every one of the survivors that I have met had a literal team of people that helped us win the FIGHT against illness. If you are serious about fighting and beating the illness that's confronting you, you too will have to assemble your own disease fighting team.

The simple truth is that you could need a team to HELP you with the most basic aspects of life. With some illnesses, you might even find that you need HELP to handle the daily cares of life. Like when you were a little child, you might need assistance to eat, bath, dress and get through all of the other day to day concerns of life. I did.

Additionally, you could go through a period where you won't be able to take on many of the personal matters that crop up while you're on the path to recovery – even things that you perfectly handled on your own before falling ill. Either you won't have the strength or you just can't be two places at the same time.

As the condition of your health changes, you may not be physically capable of caring for yourself the way you once did. Even if it is just for a temporary time, circumstances may seriously require that someone else handle life's task for you. It's the team that you've built that will come to your aid and HELP you to get through these trying times.

Speaking for me, I wouldn't have even gotten into treatment for the illness that attacked me if it were not for HELP. Like a typical man, after a year of fleeting symptoms I had still managed to avoid getting myself to the doctor to find out what was ailing me.

Even when circumstances forced me into the ER, whether out of fear or just plain stupidity, I still attempted to put off receiving the medical attention that I so obviously needed. I even brushed off a hard working nurse who had just expended a great deal of effort lining up a special package of care for me.

This wonderful lady put together a team of doctors, a private room at a great hospital, with all of the state of the art equipment that was needed to diagnose and treat my condition; with a professional medical transport team to get me there, with my insurance agreeing to allow 100% of the cost to be billed to them.

After spending three days of her professional life pulling all of this together, I looked this lady dead in the eye and said, *"I am going to go home and deal with this matter at a later time."* In typical male fashion, I attempted to decline this offer of excellent care and put off giving doctors a chance to address the growing health crisis that was glaring at me.

In that moment it took the HELP of my wife to talk me down off of the ledge and get me headed for that new hospital and into treatment. At that moment she stepped in for me and made the decision that I couldn't or wouldn't make for myself.

Thank **God** that at that moment I knew that there are times when we all need to let others take the lead and guide us in our decision making. Scripture even teaches that sometimes we need to allow others to guide us on our path where it says, *"Trust in the Lord with all your heart and lean not on your own understanding."* Proverbs 3:5. Thank **God** that at that moment, I trusted my wife and didn't lean on my own understanding.

Additionally, during my battle with multiple myeloma, my wife wore a host of hats and in the process played a major role in my recovery. She truly was my "Everything" – my spirit lifter, my filter, my encourager, my caretaker, my business partner & manager, my prayer partner, my enforcer/protector and she even assumed the role as our household's primary bread winner.

Considering all of the vital roles that she played, there's no way that I get through this crisis without her. She truly was the heart and soul of my ***"Illness Fighting Team."***

In addition, I had the HELP of a group of individuals that gave me the ability to focus 100% of my being on beating the cancer that attacked me. From my sons and my younger brother, to a few good friends and my doctor and his staff, I had a team that gave me the best chance of beating illness.

Thanks to my family and friends, I had the chance to take a break from the everyday cares of life and be 100% present to pursue the healing miracle that I needed. And thanks to my doctor and his staff, I had access to the type of world class medical care that allowed me to win that FIGHT.

I was told early on by my doctor that many people lose their FIGHT against illness because they simply never truly wage the FIGHT against it. They never show up for the FIGHT because they allow the cares and busy-ness of their life to get in the way of their pursuit of healing.

It's easily understandable why some people stricken with illness make this mistake. Life is certainly demanding. It's demanding before illness and those demands don't disappear when major illness interrupts your life.

There is no doubt that having to fight a serious illness is a major inconvenience. But still to beat it you have to avoid letting the spirit of inconvenience get the best of you and present yourself for the FIGHT. I have no doubt that I found healing largely because I did that and I was able to make finding it my sole focus when the moment called for it.

A large part of me doing that was building a team of people to HELP me make beating cancer my sole focus. Now building your own team of helpers will allow you to be present for the FIGHT of your life. And, that will give you the best chance to beat the illness that is confronting you as well. Trust me on that.

If you have a loving mate who cares about you, trust them with your care. Give him/her the authority to make the decisions that you won't or can't make for yourself.

If you have great family members and friends, get them involve. If you haven't already done so, find a caring and professional doctor. Lean on these people in this time of great need.

Trust their judgment in matters where fear or stubbornness might get the best of you. Let them lead you in areas where you may not be strong enough alone to make the right decisions concerning your pursuit of healing.

Deputize those who are in your corner to play a role in helping you manage your life so you can be present to pursue your healing. Check your pride and your ego at the door. Humble yourself and ask for the HELP and support that you need to beat illness.

Many people think humbling oneself is an act of weakness. In truth, by humbling yourself and submitting yourself to your own illness fighting team you are actually stepping into power.

Scripture teaches that we avail ourselves of power that we could never possess when we go it alone.

Ecclesiastes 4:9-10 says, *"Two are better than one, because they have a good return for their labor: If either of them falls down, one can HELP the other up. But pity anyone who falls and has no one to HELP them up."*

To be sure, having the power of two on your side as you FIGHT that illness makes it a whole lot easier for you to win.

Also, truly partner with your doctor and his medical team. Also partner with the cast of medical professionals and facilities that support your doctor in waging the FIGHT against the illness you're battling.

From a practical standpoint, it's this team that will avail you of the medicines, treatments and procedures that you will need to take down the disease that has attacked you and heal your body.

And, from a psychological standpoint, it's these efforts to FIGHT back against the illness that will give you the comfort that can only come from knowing that someone is on the job and something is being done to heal you and save your life.

Without those efforts it's pretty hard to keep in good spirits. It's even harder to keep your mind free of stress and worry over the situation. Again, almost to a person, the people who I knew who lost their FIGHT to illness had doctors who failed to give them this assurance.

In the end, this lack of assurance made the patient feel as though they were losing to illness or as if they could never beat it.

Put God On Your illness Fighting Team

Lastly, don't forget to put **God** on your team. For many people, myself included, *He* is the head of the team. But I am aware that some people don't have an active relationship with the **Creator**, just as many people have different concepts of **God**.

I'm not here to tell you what to believe. However I can tell you that every one of the survivors of major illness that I have had the good fortune to meet spoke of having an active relationship with **God**.

Each one saw *Him* as a big part of their illness fighting team and the main reason why they were able to overcome the illness they were fighting. I can also tell you without a doubt that almost to a person, the people who I personally knew who lost their fight had the exact opposite relationship to **God**.

Either these people had no active relationship with *Him*. Or, they were a non-believer all together. I'll let you interpret those facts how you see fit, as I am just the messenger.

Another truth is that it is in trying times like fighting a serious illness that many people come to their relationship with their **Creator**. Or, they strengthen a relationship that they already have.

Whichever case yours may be, the key thing is just that you add **God** to the team. In fact, scripture says that in building your team, you can automatically invite **God** to join you in your illness fighting efforts when it says,

"For where two or three gather in my name, there am I with them." Matthew 18:20.

So if you will just come together in *His* name as you FIGHT for your life, *He* promises that *He* will be there with you. That truly is bringing *His* might to the FIGHT.

If you personally need to come into relationship with **God**, in the back of this book I will share what I believe and show you how to invite **God** into your life right now.

Otherwise, to close out this program let me offer a quick list of the positions that I filled on my championship *Illness Fighting Team*.

Members of Your Illness Fighting Team
(In my experience, these teammates can HELP you beat illness.)

Lead Doctor – Doctor you trust to lead your medical FIGHT.
Lead Caretaker – Person who provides your day to day care.
Business Manager – Person handling personal & medical business.
Spirit Lifter – Person that keeps you smiling & laughing.
Shield / Filter – Person controlling what people / matters you see.

Encourager – Person heaping encouragement on you as you FIGHT.
Prayer Partner – Person who studies the word & prays with you.
Prayer Warrior – Person who knows the word & prays for you.
Enforcer / Protector – Person keeping your life / day drama free.
Bread Winner / Backer – Person keeping home afloat financially.
Time Machine – Person linking you to the old world.

It's worth saying again that each of these people must believe in your ability and mission to FIGHT and BEAT illness, just as you do. The mission of these teammates is to support you in your pursuit of healing. They are there to keep your spirits up, keep your mind off of that illness or what you may be going through at a given moment and you physically, mentally and financially free to pursue that healing.

If at any point anyone of these people ceases to fulfill those roles, he / she has to be relieved of their duties and a new person selected for the role. The key goal here is that you assemble a team of people to insulate you from the day to day distractions of life that keep a person fighting illness from finding healing.

Finally, it should go without saying that it is likely that a person in your life / inner circle will fulfill multiple roles on your team – the only caveat being that you be careful not to burn that person out in the process. In this case, more HELP is better, as from my experience there is plenty of work to go around.

What's important is that you invest the time and effort to get the roles filled. You can and should also add any other roles that you feel you need to round out your own team.

YOU Can Beat Cancer With FAITH Too!

"YOUR FAITH HAS MADE YOU WELL..."

"AND HE SAID TO HER, "DAUGHTER, YOUR FAITH HAS MADE YOU WELL, GO IN PEACE AND BE HEALED OF YOUR ILLNESS."

— MARK 5:34

So there you have a glimpse of the FAITH that I and many others have APPLIED to the FIGHT against a major illness.

F = Decide to FIGHT back!

A = Keep a positive, "Can Do" ATTITUDE!

I = Know your INSPIRATION & get the right INFORMATION!

T = Give yourself TIME to heal & Recover!

H = Get HELP to FIGHT & Beat illness!

At the end of the day my FAITH was the greatest part of how I BEAT cancer. If you will APPLY your FAITH in these 5 ways, you will give yourself the best chance to BEAT the illness that is standing in front of you. Just like me and all the survivors I have met BEAT illness.

In closing, let me leave you with this question, *"Is anything too hard for **God**?"*

This question was posed in scripture by both man and ***God Himself***. In both cases the question was prefaced with an accounting of the fact that *He* has created ALL that makes up this world and every living thing in it.

Therefore if **God** created you, doesn't it stand to reason that *He* can give you the power to heal? Scripture says, *"I will give you back your health and heal your wounds," says the LORD."* Jeremiah 30:17.

By this scripture, that is the promise of **God** for sure. Scripture teaches us that it is with our FAITH that we receive the promises of **God**. Just as it teaches that,

*"**God** has given each of us the measure of FAITH."* Romans 12:3.

I believe it is with that FAITH that we move *His* hand. It is by APPLYING that FAITH that you bring *Him* into the affairs of your lives. It is with that FAITH that you unleash the healing power of the universe on the illness that you are fighting to beat.

It's worth remembering that scripture also says that, **"With man this is impossible, but with God ALL THINGS ARE POSSIBLE"** Matthew 19:26.

It might be worthwhile to remember this when some man tries to tell you that you beating illness seems impossible, or especially when you start to feel like you beating that illness is impossible.

You might do well to remember that the illness that you are facing at this moment is part of the **"ALL THINGS"** that that scripture is talking about.

Stay mindful of this fact so you don't underestimate your power to beat illness and so that you don't speak your demise. And, most importantly, so that you don't count yourself out and accept defeat, permanent disability or even death as your fate.

Remember scripture says that, *"Death and Life are in the power of **YOUR** tongue."* No matter what the prognosis says, no matter what the doctor says, you have the right to **"SPEAK LIFE TO YOUR LIFE!"**

Remember, 8 doctors agreed that I wouldn't live to see 2013 and that I would never walk again, no matter how long I lived.

But I didn't believe that and I never allowed those sentiments into my ears and my body. I knew the power of the FAITH that **God** gave me.

And instead of believing their pessimistic views and speaking the doom they saw in my future over my life, I APPLIED MY FAITH and *"Spoke Life To My Life."* In the end,

I BEAT CANCER WITH **FAITH** & **YOU** CAN TOO!!!

Get the book that will UNLEASH your FAITH!!!

FAITH (APPLIED)

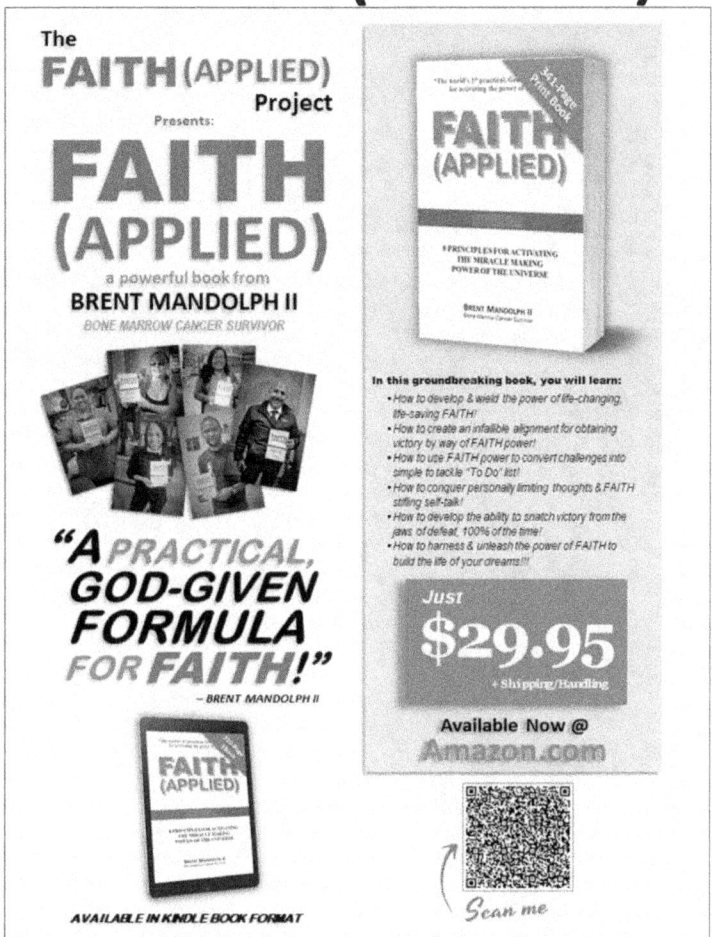

In "FAITH (APPLIED)" I will share the powerful 8 principle FAITH formula that the *Creator* revealed to me 25 years ago – wisdom that I have successfully used to activate the miracle-making power of the universe, time and again. This power has allowed me to conquer several major crisis, most notably, late stage bone marrow cancer and paralysis.

The Four Fundamental Truths of Your Recovery

– *The Four Fundamental Truths of Your Recovery: Confessing your FAITH in God's power to heal and restore you!*

Operating in FAITH works no matter what the crisis, assuming we stay in FAITH. When I first got home from the hospital, even before I could get out of the bed I assessed my situation and knew that I would need to find a way to keep the FAITH as I sought my healing. I created a detailed confession of FAITH called, *The Four Fundamental Truths of My Recovery* to help me do that.

Instead of focusing on where I was in this challenging moment, I used this confession to focus myself on the distance that I needed to travel to get back to the level of health and mobility that I enjoyed before cancer. I also used it to keep myself clear on both the progress I was making and the physical and mental things that I needed to do to make the journey back to full health.

Sticking with this confession no matter where I was in the moment has continually led me to new levels of physical, mental and emotional well-being. The example below reflects the outcome of my most recent checkups. These checkups involve me being checked from head to toe, i.e., blood work, MRI's and P.E.T. scans.

All of these test combined serve both as an early warning system and scientific confirmation for my doctors of exactly where I stand in relationship to my healing and restoration from cancer.

While I may be content to draw my own confirmation of my recovery from my FAITH, these men and women of medicine prefer to get theirs from the sciences that they have been schooled in, and that's just fine by me.

If anything, the great reports that they get back only serve to confirm the faithfulness of ***God*** in keeping his promise to heal and restore me from cancer. In turn, this also serves to bolster my willingness to continue to stand in FAITH until the day that my full health is restored.

Planned with an eye out towards both my medical and physical condition in the moment and my own recovery goals, the written confession looks like this:

SURVIVOR

The 4 Fundamental Truths of My Recovery
(To be read aloud and visualized daily)

1. – As a result of the medicines, treatments and nutritional support that I've received, this disease is placed into permanent remission, any & all growths, both new ones and those that were housed in my body have now stopped, shrunk and have disappeared from my body. (100% true as of December 18th, 2019 – per Dr. Farjami.)

(I am free of pain, presence and bodily constriction – free to enjoy my normal range of motion and mobility – I can sleep comfortably on my sides and my stomach without stressing my back, I can carry out my field marketing activities and my field recruiting and client meetings without stressing my feet and legs. (85% true as of January 1st, 2020)

2. – As my bones were being cleansed of this disease, new stronger bones were quickly growing back and taking the place of the disease-weakened bones that once existed. (100% true as of December 18th, 2019 – per Dr. Farjami.)

(I am free of the risk of breaking bones, injuring myself or causing paralysis of any kind, especially through the carrying out of my basic daily activities, sleeping on my sides or through engaging in light weight lifting / toning exercises.)

3. – Physically, I have regained near complete bodily strength, I have fluidity in and normal functional use of my lower body – i.e., my legs, the soles of my feet and my knee joints. I am now working to regain full functional use of my full core, i.e., my back & stomach muscles.

Overall, I am healthy and while I must be careful not to put stress or strain on my feet or my back, I must avoid pandering to them and being needlessly inactive because of them. (100% true as of December 18th, 2019 – per Dr. Farjami.)

(I can stand & walk comfortably & normally without causing my feet pain the next day, I am free to resume my ideal daily regimen and 30-hour weekly work schedule. I can also ramp up my full muscular rehabilitation/toning & my weight loss program. (100% true as of January 1st, 2020)

4. – I have now fully reversed the condition of neuropathy and regained normal nerve sensation, feeling and function in my hands and feet. The soles of my feet, the front of my feet & toes, my hands are all back to normal. My back & sides are free of pain, discomfort and spasms. With all things considered, I feel normal in all ways from head to toe and all places in between. (80% true as of January 1st, 2020)

(I am fully restored to the level of health, wellness and personal mobility that I enjoyed before being stricken with this disease. Now being fully healed, I am off of all medications and treatments. I have suffered no lasting or lingering side effects from taking the medications and going through the treatments that were used to heal me and make me whole again. (75% true as of January 1st, 2020)

To GOD be the glory for my Recovery & Restoration!!!

In Jesus name, AMEN!!! **Last updated, January 1st, 2020**

Needless to say, the first version of this confession of my FAITH in the healing power of ***God*** would have acknowledged the fact that after being bedridden for the 12 previous weeks, I was totally weak physically, couldn't sit up erect and could nowhere near stand, much less think of getting out of the bed and walking.

Having started from that place, to be where I am now, more than 7 years later reveals just how powerful a force FAITH is and just how far ***God*** has brought me back from the brink of a true health nightmare.

True to the spirit of FAITH that we have already talked about, I used this template to give consideration to all of the aspects that I needed to focus on in my push towards recovery and to solicit everything that I would need to get there from the ***Creator***. I now offer its example to you in the hopes that you too will use it to focus your mind on the healing and restoration that you both deserve and desire.

You can email me at: ***Template@winwithfaith.com*** to get a fill in the blank copy that will allow you to create your own *"Four Fundamentals of Recovery"* confession of FAITH.

A Personal Message for the Reader

Thank you for taking the time to read *FAITH (APPLIED)*. It's my hope that this wisdom will do for your life, all of the great things that using it has done for my life. This truly is powerful wisdom from above. But to be clear, it is not my claim that these principles alone are the source of the miracles that they make possible. Nor is it my claim that you or I are the source of the miracles that we might obtain through their use.

Hebrews 12:2 says that, Jesus Christ is the author and finisher of our faith. I must state emphatically that my faith is in my Lord and savior, Jesus Christ and the *God* that is his and our *Creator*.

Romans 12:3 says that, the *Creator* has given each one of us the measure of faith. If you have never established a personal relationship with your *Creator*, there is no greater way to get the power of *FAITH (APPLIED)* flowing in your life.

John 14:6 says that there is only one way to the Father. It is through a personal relationship with Jesus Christ. If you have never given your life to Jesus, no single act will ever do more for you in this life or in the after life to come. If you haven't yet established a relationship with Jesus, there is no better time than the present moment to do it!!!

Will you say this simple prayer?

Dear Jesus,

I know I'm a sinner and I need a savior. I believe You are the Son of God, that You died, paying the price for my sins, and rose again. I ask You to come into my life now. I now receive You as my Lord and Savior.

If you have said this simple prayer, know that you have now accepted *Jesus* as your Lord and Savior and all the angels in heaven are rejoicing! Let me both congratulate and welcome you to the Christian family! You have taken a powerful step to unleash the real and true power of *FAITH (APPLIED)* in your life.

Now get in a Christ-centered, Bible-based, Faith-centered church in your area. Most importantly, from this day forward know that *God* is real! *God* is still here! *God* is still involved in the lives of his children today! And, through *FAITH (APPLIED)*, *God* is still your personal miracle maker!

Brent Mandolph II

www.ingramcontent.com/pod-product-compliance
Lightning Source LLC
Chambersburg PA
CBHW070826220526
45466CB00002B/767